Table Of Contents

Chapter 1: The Quest for Wellness

Understanding Global Wellness

Understanding Global Wellness encompasses a rich tapestry of practices, beliefs, and lifestyles that contribute to health across different cultures. This journey through the world's healthiest populations reveals not only the physical aspects of wellness but also the profound connections between mind, body, and spirit. From the serene mountain villages of Japan to the vibrant coastal communities of the Mediterranean, each culture offers unique insights and lessons that can inspire our own wellness journeys.

The concept of wellness transcends mere absence of disease; it embodies a holistic approach to life. Traditional fermented foods, for instance, are a cornerstone of many cultures known for their longevity and vitality. In places like South Korea, kimchi is not just a side dish but a vital source of probiotics that promote gut health. Similarly, the consumption of kefir in the Caucasus region highlights the importance of these ancient food practices. By embracing these time-honored traditions, we can nurture our gut microbiomes, which play a crucial role in our overall health and well-being.

Sustainable living practices are another vital component of global wellness. Communities that prioritize harmony with nature often experience enhanced physical and mental health. For example, the Maasai of East Africa embody a sustainable lifestyle rooted in their deep connection to the land. Their diet, rich in natural foods and low in processed ingredients, reflects an understanding of balance and respect for the environment. This philosophy teaches us that our well-being is intricately linked to the health of our planet, inspiring us to adopt more sustainable habits in our daily lives.

Moreover, the social fabric of healthy communities cannot be overlooked. Cultures that emphasize strong family ties and social networks tend to enjoy better health outcomes. In Mediterranean societies, communal meals and gatherings foster connections that enhance emotional well-being. These social interactions not only provide support but also contribute to a sense of belonging, which is essential for mental health. By cultivating our own supportive networks, we can mirror this aspect of global wellness in our lives.

Ultimately, understanding global wellness encourages us to embrace a diverse array of practices and philosophies that can enrich our own lives. By exploring the healthiest cultures around the world, we gain valuable insights into nutrition, sustainability, and community. This knowledge empowers us to make informed choices, not only for our personal health but also for the well-being of our planet and future generations. As we embark on this journey, let us remain open to the wisdom of different cultures, allowing their experiences to inspire us toward a healthier, more vibrant life.

Defining Health Across Cultures

Health is a multifaceted concept that transcends mere absence of illness, varying significantly across cultures and societies. In some cultures, health is viewed as a harmonious balance between body, mind, and spirit, while in others, it is deeply intertwined with community and social relationships. For instance, Indigenous cultures often emphasize the interconnectedness of all living things, seeing health as a reflection of one's relationship with nature and the community. This holistic approach encourages individuals to nurture their surroundings and foster strong social ties, illustrating that health is not solely a personal endeavor but a collective one.

In many Asian cultures, the principles of Traditional Chinese Medicine exemplify a unique understanding of health that incorporates balance and energy flow. Concepts such as Yin and Yang and Qi illustrate that health is about maintaining equilibrium in all aspects of life. The practice of Tai Chi, for example, not only promotes physical fitness but also cultivates mental clarity and emotional stability. This emphasis on balance highlights the importance of integrating physical, mental, and spiritual health, a perspective that resonates with the growing global interest in holistic wellness practices.

The Mediterranean region offers another enlightening perspective on health, with its emphasis on diet, lifestyle, and social interaction. The Mediterranean diet, rich in fruits, vegetables, whole grains, and healthy fats, is celebrated not just for its nutritional value but also for its role in fostering community. Shared meals and social gatherings are central to this lifestyle, illustrating how cultural practices can enhance well-being. This communal aspect serves as a reminder that health is often a shared experience, deeply rooted in the social fabric of daily life.

Traditional fermented foods, prevalent in cultures worldwide, also play a vital role in defining health. From kimchi in Korea to sauerkraut in Germany, these foods are celebrated not only for their probiotic benefits but also for their cultural significance. They represent a connection to heritage and tradition, often passed down through generations. The consumption of these foods emphasizes the importance of gut health, illustrating how cultural practices can have profound implications for physical health. This connection between tradition and well-being highlights the value of incorporating time-honored practices into contemporary wellness approaches.

Ultimately, defining health across cultures invites us to reconsider our own perceptions of wellness. It encourages us to look beyond individualistic models and embrace a more interconnected understanding of health. By exploring diverse cultural practices, we can uncover valuable insights into sustainable living and its effects on well-being. Each culture presents a unique tapestry of beliefs, practices, and traditions that can inspire us to cultivate a more holistic approach to our health, emphasizing the importance of community, tradition, and balance in our pursuit of wellness.

The Importance of a Holistic Approach

In a world increasingly driven by specialization and compartmentalization, the importance of a holistic approach to wellness emerges as a beacon of hope. This perspective encourages us to view health not merely as the absence of disease but as a dynamic interplay of physical, mental, emotional, and spiritual well-being. Cultures that have thrived for centuries often embrace holistic practices, recognizing the interconnectedness of all life aspects. As we explore the healthiest populations globally, we uncover profound insights into how a comprehensive approach can lead to vibrant living and longevity.

Traditional fermented foods are a cornerstone of this holistic philosophy, playing a vital role in the health of many cultures. These foods, rich in probiotics, enhance gut health, which is increasingly recognized as essential for overall wellness. The relationship between a healthy gut and a strong immune system, improved mood, and even better cognitive function highlights the significance of these ancient practices. By integrating fermented foods into our diets, we honor the wisdom of generations past while fostering a deeper connection to our bodies and the natural world around us.

Sustainable living also embodies the essence of a holistic approach, intertwining environmental health with personal well-being. Cultures that prioritize sustainability often cultivate a profound respect for nature, understanding that our health is inextricably linked to the ecosystems we inhabit. By adopting practices that promote environmental stewardship—such as organic farming, mindful consumption, and waste reduction—we not only enhance our health but also contribute to a more balanced planet. This symbiotic relationship between personal wellness and environmental health invites us to consider how our choices impact not just ourselves but also future generations.

Moreover, the holistic approach encourages us to embrace the emotional and spiritual dimensions of health. Mindfulness, meditation, and communal practices are prevalent in the healthiest cultures, reinforcing the idea that well-being extends beyond the physical realm. These practices foster resilience, enhance emotional intelligence, and cultivate a sense of belonging, which are vital in navigating the complexities of modern life. By nurturing our mental and spiritual health, we build a foundation that supports our physical health, creating a comprehensive model for living well.

In conclusion, embracing a holistic approach to wellness opens doors to a richer, more fulfilling life. By learning from the healthiest cultures around the globe, we can incorporate traditional wisdom, sustainable practices, and emotional resilience into our daily routines. This journey towards holistic well-being not only transforms our health but also connects us to the broader tapestry of life, reminding us that true wellness is a shared experience, woven together by our choices, actions, and the love we cultivate within ourselves and our communities.

Chapter 2: The Healthiest Nations on Earth

Japan: The Secret to Longevity

Japan is often celebrated for its remarkable health outcomes and high life expectancy, which has intrigued researchers and wellness enthusiasts alike. The secret to longevity in Japan lies not only in genetics but also in a harmonious blend of traditional practices, dietary habits, and a deep-rooted cultural appreciation for well-being. This vibrant culture nurtures the body and spirit, offering valuable lessons for individuals seeking to enhance their health and longevity.

At the heart of Japanese longevity is the traditional diet, which is rich in fresh, seasonal ingredients. The Japanese cuisine emphasizes the consumption of vegetables, fish, and fermented foods, all of which provide essential nutrients and promote gut health. Staples like miso, pickled vegetables, and natto are not just culinary delights; they are powerhouses of probiotics that support digestive health and boost the immune system. This focus on natural, whole foods creates a balanced diet that nourishes the body and fosters vitality.

Moreover, the Japanese practice of "Hara Hachi Bu," the principle of eating until one is 80% full, plays a crucial role in maintaining a healthy weight and preventing chronic diseases. This mindful approach to eating encourages individuals to savor their meals, promoting a deeper connection with food and an appreciation for moderation. By cultivating awareness around portion sizes and the quality of food consumed, the Japanese exemplify how conscious eating can lead to improved health outcomes.

Sustainable living is another cornerstone of Japanese culture that contributes to overall well-being. The Japanese have a profound respect for nature, which is reflected in their daily habits and community practices. Urban gardens, local markets, and a commitment to reducing waste not only enhance environmental health but also foster a sense of community and belonging. This connection to nature and commitment to sustainability encourages a lifestyle that supports mental and emotional health, creating a holistic approach to wellness.

In summary, Japan's secret to longevity is a tapestry woven from mindful eating, a rich repository of traditional foods, and a deep respect for the environment. As the world seeks answers to the challenges of modern living, the Japanese way of life offers profound insights into achieving health and well-being. By adopting these principles, individuals everywhere can cultivate a lifestyle that honors both their bodies and the planet, paving the way to a longer, healthier life.

Mediterranean Magic: Greece and Italy

The sun-kissed coasts of Greece and Italy are not merely idyllic vacation spots; they embody a unique blend of culture, tradition, and wellness that has been cherished for centuries. Both countries boast a rich history of healthful living that melds seamlessly with their culinary practices, offering a lifestyle that celebrates balance and nourishment. The Mediterranean diet, with its emphasis on fresh vegetables, whole grains, legumes, and healthy fats, has been heralded as a cornerstone of wellness. This lifestyle promotes not just physical health, but also emotional and social well-being, creating a holistic approach to life that is as enchanting as the landscapes themselves.

In Greece, the tradition of communal meals reflects the deep social ties that contribute to overall well-being. Families and friends gather to share dishes prepared with locally sourced ingredients, emphasizing the importance of connection and community. Traditional fermented foods, such as yogurt and olives, are staples of the Greek diet, packed with probiotics that support gut health. This age-old practice of fermentation not only enhances flavor but also provides a wealth of health benefits, resonating with modern understandings of nutrition. The Greeks understand that food is not just sustenance; it is a vehicle for social interaction and emotional fulfillment.

Italy, too, boasts its own magical culinary traditions, where meals are celebrated as an art form rather than a mere necessity. The Italian approach to food is deeply rooted in the concept of "la dolce vita," a philosophy that encourages savoring life's pleasures, including food. The Italian diet is rich in fresh produce, legumes, and whole grains, complemented by olive oil and moderate portions of wine. This diet has been linked to reduced rates of chronic diseases and a higher quality of life. The Italians' commitment to sustainability—favoring local and seasonal ingredients—further enhances their health and well-being, proving that caring for the environment is intrinsically tied to personal wellness.

Sustainable living in both Greece and Italy extends beyond dietary choices; it encompasses a lifestyle that prioritizes connection to nature, community, and tradition. In rural villages and coastal towns, you will find practices that respect the land and its resources, ensuring that future generations can enjoy the same bounty. This respect for nature is evident in the artisanal production of foods, from hand-picked olives to organic vegetables, reinforcing the idea that wellness is a shared responsibility. The slower pace of life in these regions encourages mindfulness, a crucial element in mitigating stress and fostering mental health.

Ultimately, the allure of Greece and Italy lies not only in their breathtaking landscapes and vibrant cultures but also in their profound understanding of wellness as a collective journey. The Mediterranean magic encapsulates a lifestyle that intertwines health, happiness, and community, inviting individuals to embrace a holistic approach to living. By learning from these cultures, we can cultivate our own practices that enhance our well-being, reminding us that true health flourishes at the intersection of nutrition, connection, and sustainability.

Nordic Wisdom: Denmark and Sweden

Nordic countries, particularly Denmark and Sweden, have long been recognized for their unique approach to wellness, combining a deep respect for nature with an emphasis on community and personal well-being. The concept of "hygge" in Denmark reflects this ethos, focusing on coziness, contentment, and an appreciation for simple pleasures. This cultural practice encourages individuals to create warm, inviting spaces and prioritize quality time with loved ones, reinforcing the idea that emotional well-being is integral to overall health. In Sweden, the concept of "lagom," meaning "just the right amount," promotes balance and moderation, urging people to seek equilibrium in their lives. Together, these philosophies foster a holistic approach to health that resonates globally.

Traditional fermented foods play a significant role in the diets of both Denmark and Sweden, contributing to gut health and overall wellness. In Denmark, the love for fermented products is evident in staples like "surdejsbrød," or sourdough bread, and "rødkål," pickled red cabbage. These foods not only enhance flavor but also support the microbiome, essential for digestion and immunity. Similarly, Sweden boasts a rich tradition of fermentation with foods like "surströmming," fermented herring, and "kefir," a fermented milk drink. These time-honored practices highlight how the preservation of food can be both a culinary delight and a pathway to improved health, underscoring the connection between diet, culture, and wellness.

Sustainable living is deeply ingrained in the lifestyles of both Danes and Swedes, profoundly affecting their overall well-being. Denmark consistently ranks as one of the world's happiest countries, in part due to its commitment to environmental sustainability. Urban planning in cities like Copenhagen promotes biking, green spaces, and accessible public transport, encouraging active lifestyles and reducing stress. Sweden, too, champions sustainability with initiatives that prioritize renewable energy, waste reduction, and organic farming. This commitment to the environment not only fosters a sense of community and shared responsibility but also enhances the quality of life for individuals, creating a healthier, more vibrant society.

The integration of nature into daily life is a cornerstone of wellness in these Nordic countries. Both Denmark and Sweden boast stunning landscapes, from the serene coastlines to lush forests, inviting inhabitants to engage with the outdoors. Outdoor activities such as hiking, cycling, and swimming in natural waters are common, promoting physical health while also offering mental rejuvenation. The Scandinavian concept of "friluftsliv," or open-air living, encourages people to embrace nature regardless of the season, reinforcing the idea that connection to the natural world is vital for emotional and physical health. This harmonious relationship with the environment nurtures resilience and fosters a profound sense of belonging.

In conclusion, Denmark and Sweden exemplify how cultural practices, traditional diets, and sustainable living converge to create a holistic approach to wellness. Their emphasis on community, balance, and connection to nature serves as an inspiration for those seeking to enhance their own well-being. The Nordic wisdom of these nations teaches us that health is not merely the absence of illness but a multi-faceted experience shaped by our choices, our environments, and our relationships. By embracing these principles, individuals around the globe can cultivate healthier, more fulfilling lives, drawing inspiration from the rich traditions and modern practices of the Nordic way of living.

The Resilience of Bhutan's Happiness

The resilience of Bhutan's happiness stands as a testament to the profound connection between culture, environment, and well-being. Nestled in the eastern Himalayas, Bhutan has gained global recognition for its unique approach to measuring success through Gross National Happiness (GNH) rather than traditional economic indicators. This philosophy reflects a deep-rooted understanding that true prosperity encompasses not just material wealth, but also the spiritual, emotional, and environmental health of its citizens. The Bhutanese people's unwavering commitment to this holistic model of happiness illustrates a powerful narrative about how well-being can thrive even in the face of modern challenges.

One of the cornerstones of Bhutan's happiness is its emphasis on sustainable living. The country has prioritized ecological preservation, with over 70 percent of its land designated as protected areas. This dedication to nature fosters a strong sense of community and stewardship among the Bhutanese people. By engaging in sustainable agricultural practices and promoting organic farming, Bhutan not only protects its biodiversity but also ensures that its citizens have access to healthy, locally sourced food. This sustainable approach to living enriches their diets and strengthens their connection to the land, contributing to both physical health and emotional well-being.

Bhutan's rich tradition of fermented foods plays a significant role in enhancing gut health and overall wellness. Dishes like ema datshi, made with locally grown chilies and cheese, showcase the unique flavors that come from traditional fermentation methods. These foods are not only beloved for their taste but also for their nutritional benefits, promoting a healthy gut microbiome that is essential for physical vitality. The Bhutanese people's commitment to preserving their culinary heritage through these time-honored practices highlights the importance of food in nurturing both body and spirit, creating a culture that celebrates the joy of eating well.

Resilience in Bhutan is also reflected in the community's approach to mental health. The Bhutanese recognize the interconnectedness of emotional well-being and societal harmony. By fostering a culture that values open dialogue about mental health, the country empowers its citizens to seek support and nurture their emotional resilience. Initiatives that promote mindfulness, meditation, and community gatherings exemplify Bhutan's understanding that happiness is a collective endeavor. This emphasis on mental wellness strengthens social bonds and creates a supportive environment that enables individuals to thrive.

In conclusion, the resilience of Bhutan's happiness serves as an inspiring model for the world. By prioritizing sustainable living, embracing traditional practices, and fostering community support, Bhutan offers valuable lessons on how to cultivate well-being in an ever-changing global landscape. As societies around the globe grapple with the challenges of modern life, Bhutan's holistic approach stands as a beacon of hope, illustrating that happiness is not merely an individual pursuit but a shared journey that can lead to a healthier, more harmonious world.

Chapter 3: Traditional Fermented Foods and Gut Health

The Science of Fermentation

The science of fermentation offers a fascinating glimpse into the intricate relationship between nature and nourishment. Fermentation, an ancient process that transforms food through the action of microorganisms, has shaped culinary traditions across the globe. From the tangy taste of kimchi in Korea to the rich flavors of sauerkraut in Germany, the diversity of fermented foods is a testament to human ingenuity in preserving and enhancing the nutritional value of our meals.

This age-old practice not only enriches our diets but also serves as a bridge connecting us to our ancestors, who relied on these techniques for sustenance, health, and survival.

At the heart of fermentation lies a complex community of microorganisms, including bacteria, yeast, and molds, that interact with food in profound ways. These tiny organisms break down sugars and starches, producing beneficial compounds such as lactic acid, alcohol, and carbon dioxide. This process not only extends the shelf life of food but also creates a host of probiotics that contribute to gut health. In cultures where fermented foods are staples, such as in Japan with miso and in Eastern Europe with kefir, people often enjoy enhanced digestion and overall well-being, showcasing the powerful impact of these foods on health.

The benefits of fermented foods extend beyond gut health. They are rich in vitamins, minerals, and bioactive compounds that bolster the immune system and promote mental clarity. For example, the fermentation process can increase the availability of nutrients, making them more accessible for absorption in the body. Cultures around the world have long recognized the importance of these foods, integrating them into their diets not merely for taste but for their vital role in maintaining health. As the world awakens to the importance of holistic wellness, the revival of fermented foods serves as a reminder of the wisdom embedded in traditional practices.

Sustainable living is another critical aspect that intertwines with the science of fermentation. Many fermented foods require minimal resources, relying instead on natural processes and local ingredients. This sustainability aligns with the growing global movement toward eco-conscious eating habits. By embracing fermentation, we not only nourish ourselves but also support local economies and reduce food waste. As we cultivate a deeper understanding of fermentation, we find ourselves engaging in a practice that honors the earth while celebrating the diverse flavors that different cultures offer.

In exploring the science of fermentation, we uncover a timeless message of resilience, creativity, and connection. The cultures that prioritize fermented foods often exhibit remarkable health outcomes, demonstrating the profound link between diet, community, and well-being. By incorporating these traditional foods into our modern lives, we can tap into a wealth of knowledge that promotes longevity and vitality. As we continue to discover and celebrate the healthiest practices from around the world, let us embrace the transformative power of fermentation, fostering not just better health for ourselves but also a sustainable future for generations to come.

Fermented Foods Around the World

Fermented foods have long been a cornerstone of culinary traditions across the globe, serving as more than just sustenance; they embody the wisdom of cultures that have thrived for centuries. From the tangy kimchi of Korea to the rich, creamy cheese of France, these foods are steeped in history and health benefits. They not only enhance flavors but also promote gut health, vital for overall well-being. As we explore the diverse landscape of fermented foods, we discover how these age-old practices contribute to the wellness of some of the healthiest populations on the planet.

In Asia, fermentation is an art form, with each country showcasing its unique techniques and flavors. In Japan, miso and natto are staples that offer not just taste but also a plethora of probiotics that support digestive health. These foods are integral to the Japanese diet, which is often cited among the healthiest in the world. Meanwhile, in Southeast Asia, the sharp and spicy flavors of fish sauce and shrimp paste highlight the importance of fermentation in enhancing the nutritional profile of meals. Such practices illustrate how traditional methods can lead to sustainable living, preserving food while nourishing communities.

Moving to Europe, fermented foods find their place in almost every culture. The Germans boast sauerkraut, a fermented cabbage dish packed with vitamins and probiotics, while the French take pride in their diverse range of cheeses, many of which undergo fermentation processes that enhance their flavor and digestibility. In Eastern Europe, kvass and kefir are cherished for their health benefits, showcasing how these delightful beverages have become part of daily life. Each of these fermented foods tells a story of resilience and adaptation, reflecting the importance of community and shared knowledge in maintaining health and traditions.

In Africa, fermentation plays a crucial role in both food preservation and health. Traditional dishes like injera, a sourdough flatbread from Ethiopia, and ogi, a fermented cereal pudding, are not only staples but also sources of vital nutrients. These foods support gut health and have been linked to improved immunity, emphasizing the connection between food practices and overall well-being. The communal aspect of preparing and sharing fermented foods fosters social ties, reminding us that health is not just an individual journey but a collective experience rooted in culture.

As we traverse the globe, the common thread that links these diverse fermented foods is their ability to promote health and sustainability. Each culture has adapted its fermentation practices to local ingredients and traditions, resulting in a rich tapestry of flavors and health benefits. By embracing these time-honored methods, we can learn valuable lessons on how to nourish our bodies and the planet. The journey into the world of fermented foods encourages us to appreciate the wisdom of our ancestors and inspires us to integrate these practices into our modern lives for a healthier future.

The Gut Microbiome: An Ecosystem Within

The gut microbiome, a complex and diverse ecosystem teeming with trillions of microorganisms, serves as a silent yet powerful contributor to our overall health and wellness. This intricate community of bacteria, viruses, fungi, and other microbes resides in our digestive tract, playing a pivotal role in processes ranging from digestion to immune function. As we delve into the rich tapestry of cultures around the world, we find that many of the healthiest populations have cultivated a profound understanding of the significance of their gut microbiome, often through traditional dietary practices that prioritize the consumption of fermented foods.

In numerous cultures, fermented foods are not merely culinary delights but are revered as essential elements of daily nutrition. From the tangy kimchi of Korea to the creamy kefir of Eastern Europe, these foods are brimming with probiotics—live microorganisms that confer health benefits when consumed in adequate amounts. The people of these regions have thrived on diets rich in these natural powerhouses, which help restore and maintain a balanced gut microbiome. This balance is crucial for preventing a myriad of health issues, from digestive disorders to mental health challenges, underscoring the wisdom embedded in these time-honored traditions.

Sustainable living practices also intertwine beautifully with the health of the gut microbiome. Many of the world's healthiest cultures emphasize a connection to nature, sourcing their food locally and seasonally. This approach not only fosters a sense of community and environmental stewardship but also enhances the nutritional quality of the food consumed. Fresh, locally sourced ingredients are more likely to be rich in prebiotics—non-digestible fibers that feed beneficial gut bacteria—supporting a thriving microbiome. This synergy between sustainable practices and gut health illuminates a path towards holistic wellness, where mindfulness in food choices promotes both personal and planetary health.

Moreover, the growing body of research highlights the profound impact of the gut microbiome on mental health, metabolism, and chronic disease prevention. The concept of the gut-brain axis illustrates how the health of our microbiome can influence our mood, cognitive function, and even our behavior. Cultures that prioritize fermented foods and sustainable eating often report lower levels of anxiety and depression, showcasing the potential of these dietary practices to enhance mental well-being. By embracing the wisdom of traditional diets, we can cultivate a deeper connection to our bodies and minds, ultimately leading to a more harmonious existence.

In conclusion, the gut microbiome stands as a testament to the intricate relationship between our health and the ecosystems we inhabit. The lessons gleaned from the healthiest cultures invite us to explore the transformative power of traditional fermented foods and sustainable living. By honoring these practices, we can nurture our gut microbiome, foster resilience against disease, and enhance our overall well-being. The journey towards wellness is not solely an individual endeavor; it is a collective movement towards a healthier future, rooted in the rich traditions that have sustained humanity for generations.

Healing Through Food: Probiotics and Prebiotics

In the vibrant tapestry of global wellness, food emerges as a powerful healer, especially through the lens of probiotics and prebiotics. Cultures around the world have long understood the profound connection between diet and health, often passing down traditions that emphasize the importance of gut health. Whether it's the tangy taste of kimchi from Korea, the creamy texture of yogurt from Greece, or the rich flavors of miso from Japan, these traditional fermented foods are not just culinary delights; they are vital components of a holistic approach to wellness. By embracing these foods, we can tap into centuries of wisdom that celebrates the role of beneficial bacteria in our bodies.

Probiotics, the live microorganisms found in fermented foods, serve as allies in our quest for optimal health. They contribute to a balanced gut microbiome, which plays a crucial role in digestion, immunity, and even mental well-being. Countries known for their healthy populations often incorporate these foods into their daily diets. In Japan, for instance, the consumption of natto, a fermented soybean dish, is linked to numerous health benefits, including improved digestion and enhanced nutrient absorption. This connection between traditional eating habits and wellness highlights the importance of nurturing our bodies with foods that support our natural processes.

On the other hand, prebiotics are the unsung heroes that feed these beneficial bacteria, allowing them to flourish. Foods rich in prebiotics, such as garlic, onions, and bananas, are essential for maintaining a thriving gut environment. Many cultures emphasize the consumption of these foods alongside their probiotic counterparts, creating a harmonious balance that promotes overall health. In Mediterranean diets, for example, the use of whole grains and plant-based ingredients not only enhances flavor but also ensures that the gut receives the nutrition it craves. This synergy between probiotics and prebiotics is a powerful testament to the wisdom embedded in traditional culinary practices.

Sustainable living is intricately linked to the consumption of probiotics and prebiotics. By choosing locally sourced, seasonal ingredients and embracing fermentation techniques, individuals can support their health while also caring for the planet. Fermented foods often have a longer shelf life, reducing waste and encouraging mindful consumption. Traditional practices, such as pickling and fermenting, have been passed down through generations as a means of preserving food and enhancing its nutritional profile. By rediscovering these methods, we not only improve our gut health but also foster a deeper connection to our food sources and the environment.

As we navigate our modern lifestyles, the lessons from cultures that prioritize gut health through food remain invaluable. By incorporating probiotics and prebiotics into our diets, we can honor these traditions and enhance our well-being. Embracing the healing power of food invites us to explore new flavors, appreciate the wisdom of our ancestors, and cultivate a sustainable approach to wellness. In doing so, we embark on a journey that celebrates the profound relationship between what we eat and how we feel, ultimately guiding us toward a healthier, more vibrant life.

Chapter 4: Sustainable Living and Its Effects on Wellbeing

The Connection Between Sustainability and Health

The connection between sustainability and health is an intricate tapestry woven through the very fabric of our existence. As we strive for a healthier life, we must embrace the relationship between our well-being and the planet's health. Cultures worldwide have long understood that nurturing the environment is essential for nurturing ourselves. From the lush rice paddies of Asia to the vibrant markets of Mediterranean villages, the wisdom of sustainable practices is evident. These practices not only provide nourishment but also foster a symbiotic relationship with nature, highlighting that our personal health is inextricably linked to the health of the Earth.

Traditional fermented foods, rich in probiotics, serve as a powerful example of this connection. Cultures that prioritize these foods, such as kimchi in Korea or sauerkraut in Germany, showcase how age-old practices of preservation also promote gut health. When we consume these nutrient-dense foods, we are not only supporting our microbiome but also participating in a sustainable cycle of food production. The fermentation process often utilizes local ingredients, minimizing transportation impact and supporting local farmers. This harmonious relationship between food production and health illustrates how mindful eating can lead to a healthier populace while simultaneously protecting our ecosystems.

Sustainable living extends beyond diet; it encompasses our lifestyle choices, including energy consumption, waste management, and transportation methods. Communities that embrace sustainability often exhibit lower rates of chronic diseases and improved mental health. Urban areas designed with green spaces and walkable neighborhoods promote physical activity and social interaction, which are vital components of overall health. By prioritizing sustainability, we create environments that enhance well-being and foster a sense of community, reminding us that we are not alone in our journey towards health.

Moreover, the practice of sustainability can inspire a deeper connection to the natural world, which has been shown to have profound effects on mental health. Nature has a unique ability to rejuvenate the spirit and calm the mind. Cultures that prioritize outdoor activities and natural surroundings, such as the Nordic countries with their emphasis on friluftsliv or "open-air living," experience lower rates of anxiety and depression. This connection to nature encourages us to appreciate the beauty around us, reinforcing the idea that our health is intertwined with the planet's vitality.

In conclusion, the synergy between sustainability and health is a call to action for individuals and communities alike. By recognizing that our choices impact not only our own well-being but also that of the environment, we can cultivate a healthier future. Embracing traditional practices, adopting sustainable lifestyles, and fostering a connection with nature can lead to a flourishing world where individuals thrive alongside the planet. As we uncover the healthiest cultures around the globe, let us draw inspiration from their wisdom and take steps towards a sustainable and healthful life.

Indigenous Practices: A Model for Modern Living

Indigenous practices, steeped in centuries of wisdom, offer profound insights into modern living. These time-honored traditions emphasize a harmonious relationship with nature, community, and self-care that resonates deeply with contemporary wellness seekers. As we navigate the complexities of urban life and modern conveniences, we can draw inspiration from the holistic approaches of Indigenous cultures that prioritize balance, sustainability, and well-being. By embracing these practices, we can foster a deeper connection to our environment and enhance our health, ultimately creating a more fulfilling lifestyle.

One of the most significant aspects of Indigenous practices is the emphasis on natural, whole foods, many of which are fermented. Traditional fermented foods, such as kimchi, sauerkraut, and various types of yogurt, have been integral to Indigenous diets around the world. These foods not only enhance gut health through probiotics but also reflect a sustainable approach to food preparation and preservation. By incorporating these nutrient-dense, fermented foods into our diets, we can nourish our bodies while honoring the traditions that have long supported community health and resilience.

Sustainable living is another cornerstone of Indigenous wisdom. Many Indigenous communities have thrived by living in harmony with their surroundings, utilizing resources in a way that respects the land and maintains ecological balance. This principle of sustainability extends to farming practices, such as crop rotation and companion planting, which promote biodiversity and soil health. By adopting these practices in our own lives, we can contribute to a more sustainable food system, reduce our ecological footprint, and cultivate a deeper appreciation for the interconnectedness of all living things.

Furthermore, Indigenous cultures often prioritize mental and emotional well-being through community connections and storytelling. Rituals, gatherings, and shared experiences create a sense of belonging that is vital for psychological health. In a world increasingly dominated by isolation and digital interactions, we can learn from these practices by fostering community ties and engaging in meaningful relationships. By sharing our stories and supporting one another, we can enhance our collective well-being and create a more nurturing environment for ourselves and future generations.

Incorporating Indigenous practices into our modern lives is not merely a nod to tradition; it is a powerful pathway to holistic wellness. As we embrace the lessons learned from these cultures, we can create a lifestyle that values health, sustainability, and community. By honoring the wisdom of Indigenous peoples, we can not only improve our own well-being but also contribute to a more balanced and resilient world. This journey toward wellness is an invitation to explore, learn, and grow, ultimately leading us to a life that resonates with the rhythms of nature and the richness of our shared human experience.

Urban Gardening: Greening Our Cities

Urban gardening is not just a trend; it is a powerful movement that is transforming the very fabric of our cities. As concrete jungles continue to expand, the need for green spaces becomes increasingly vital. Urban gardening offers a pathway to reconnect with nature, promoting not only environmental sustainability but also individual and community well-being. By cultivating gardens in our backyards, rooftops, and even on balconies, we are infusing life and color into our urban landscapes, creating havens of tranquility amidst the hustle and bustle of city life.

The benefits of urban gardening extend far beyond aesthetics. Engaging with plants fosters a sense of responsibility and connection to the Earth. Individuals who participate in urban gardening often report reduced stress levels, greater feelings of happiness, and improved mental health. The act of nurturing plants offers a therapeutic escape, allowing urban dwellers to step away from their screens and immerse themselves in nature. As we cultivate our gardens, we cultivate our well-being, creating a sanctuary that nourishes both our bodies and our souls.

Moreover, urban gardens play a crucial role in promoting sustainability. By growing our food locally, we reduce our carbon footprint and minimize the environmental impact associated with transporting goods over long distances. This practice not only ensures fresher produce but also fosters a sense of community among neighbors who share a passion for sustainable living. Urban gardening encourages people to exchange knowledge, resources, and even homegrown produce, weaving a rich tapestry of connection and collaboration that strengthens the bonds within our communities.

As urban gardening continues to flourish, it also serves as a powerful educational tool. Schools and community organizations can harness the power of gardens to teach children and adults alike about nutrition, ecology, and the importance of biodiversity. By instilling a love for gardening in future generations, we are nurturing a culture that values healthful eating and environmental stewardship. This knowledge is vital for fostering healthier lifestyles, as individuals learn the benefits of consuming fresh, organic produce and the joy of growing their own food.

Ultimately, urban gardening represents a collective journey toward greening our cities and enriching our lives. As we dig our hands into the soil, we connect with our roots—both literally and metaphorically. This movement is a testament to humanity's resilience and creativity in the face of urban challenges. By embracing the potential of urban gardening, we can transform not only our neighborhoods but also our health, happiness, and harmony with the planet. Together, we can cultivate a greener future, one garden at a time.

Minimalism and Mental Clarity

Minimalism, at its core, is about stripping away the unnecessary to reveal the essential. In a world saturated with distractions, the philosophy of minimalism emerges as a beacon of clarity. When we embrace this lifestyle, we begin to notice a profound shift in our mental landscape. By prioritizing what truly matters and letting go of the excess, we can cultivate a sense of peace and focus that is often elusive amidst the noise of modern life. This journey toward mental clarity not only enhances our personal well-being but also aligns harmoniously with the sustainable practices of the healthiest cultures around the globe.

Countries that champion minimalism often exhibit remarkable mental clarity among their populations. For instance, the Japanese concept of "Ikigai," which encourages individuals to discover their purpose, is a minimalist approach to living that fosters contentment and mental sharpness. This pursuit of meaning leads to a profound understanding of what is vital in life, enabling individuals to cultivate relationships, hobbies, and work that resonate deeply with their values. As we learn from such cultures, adopting a minimalist mindset can help us sift through the clutter, allowing us to focus on what enriches our lives, ultimately leading to greater happiness and fulfillment.

The link between minimalism and mental clarity extends beyond personal well-being; it also plays a pivotal role in our physical health. A simplified lifestyle often encourages healthier choices, such as consuming traditional fermented foods. These foods are not only beneficial for gut health but also mirror the principles of minimalism by relying on natural ingredients and time-honored preparation methods. When we simplify our diets and choose foods that are nourishing and sustainable, we create a symbiotic relationship between our mental clarity and physical well-being. This holistic approach echoes the practices of cultures that prioritize health through simplicity, reminding us that what we consume impacts both our minds and our bodies.

Embracing minimalism can also inspire sustainable living practices that contribute to environmental well-being. By reducing our consumption and focusing on quality over quantity, we not only declutter our lives but also lessen our ecological footprint. Many of the world's healthiest societies understand this connection deeply, living in ways that honor both their bodies and the planet. As we adopt a minimalist mindset, we become more attuned to our surroundings, fostering a sense of connection to nature that further enhances our mental clarity. This awareness can lead to a more purposeful existence, where our actions reflect our values and contribute positively to the world.

Ultimately, the journey toward minimalism and mental clarity is a transformative one. It challenges us to rethink our relationship with material possessions, our diets, and our lifestyles. As we cultivate this mindset, we find that the path to wellness is not solely about what we acquire, but rather what we choose to release. By embracing simplicity, we invite mental clarity into our lives, aligning ourselves with the healthiest cultures around the globe that exemplify balance, sustainability, and authentic living. In this pursuit, we discover that true wealth lies in the richness of our experiences and the depth of our connections, both with ourselves and the world around us.

Chapter 5: Integrating Wellness Practices into Daily Life

Mindfulness and Meditation: Eastern Influences

Mindfulness and meditation, rooted in ancient Eastern traditions, have captivated the modern world with their profound impact on mental and physical well-being. These practices, originating from cultures steeped in spirituality and holistic health, offer a sanctuary for the busy, often chaotic lives that many lead today. In countries like India and Japan, mindfulness is not merely a practice but a way of life, intricately woven into the fabric of society. By embracing these ancient techniques, individuals can cultivate a deeper connection to themselves and their surroundings, fostering a sense of peace and clarity in an increasingly fast-paced world.

The essence of mindfulness lies in its ability to anchor individuals in the present moment. This practice encourages a heightened awareness of thoughts, feelings, and sensations, enabling people to experience life more fully. In Buddhist traditions, mindfulness is an integral component of meditation, aimed at cultivating compassion and understanding. As people begin to practice mindfulness, they often discover how to navigate stress and anxiety, leading to improved mental health. This journey inward not only enhances personal well-being but also nurtures a sense of interconnectedness with others and the environment, promoting a sustainable lifestyle that resonates with the global movement towards holistic health.

Meditation, another cornerstone of Eastern wellness philosophies, serves as a powerful tool for self-discovery and emotional balance. Techniques such as Zen meditation and Transcendental Meditation have gained widespread popularity, transcending cultural boundaries. These practices encourage individuals to quiet their minds, delve into their inner selves, and cultivate a profound sense of inner peace. Scientific studies have documented the myriad benefits of meditation, including reduced stress levels, improved concentration, and enhanced emotional resilience. As more people around the globe turn to these techniques, they find not only personal transformation but also a shared commitment to healthier, more mindful living.

The influence of mindfulness and meditation extends beyond individual practices; they have inspired a global movement towards wellness that embraces sustainable living. In countries where these practices are prevalent, there is often a strong emphasis on the balance between mind, body, and nature. Traditional practices, such as the Japanese concept of "shinrin-yoku," or forest bathing, highlight the healing power of nature and the importance of environmental stewardship. By integrating mindfulness into daily routines, individuals can foster a deeper appreciation for the natural world, promoting sustainable choices that benefit both personal health and the planet.

As we explore the intersection of Eastern influences on mindfulness and meditation with the quest for wellness, it becomes clear that these practices offer valuable lessons for a healthier future. They remind us of the importance of being present, nurturing our mental and emotional well-being, and living in harmony with nature. By embracing these ancient teachings, individuals can unlock the potential for transformative change, not only within themselves but also in the broader context of their communities and the world. In the journey toward wellness, mindfulness and meditation stand as guiding lights, illuminating the path to a more balanced and fulfilling life.

Physical Activity: Lessons from Active Cultures

Physical activity is a cornerstone of wellness that transcends borders and cultures. In examining the lifestyles of some of the healthiest populations around the globe, we discover that physical activity is not merely a structured routine but an integral part of daily life. In cultures where movement is woven into the fabric of existence, people engage in activities that promote strength, flexibility, and endurance, often without the need for a gym. For instance, the people of Okinawa, Japan, embrace a philosophy of "ikigai," where purposeful living encourages them to remain active well into their later years. They cultivate gardens, walk daily, and partake in traditional dances, demonstrating that movement can be a joyful expression rather than a chore.

In addition to Okinawa, the vitality of the Mediterranean lifestyle showcases the benefits of physical activity intermingled with social connections. In villages across Greece and Italy, community gatherings often revolve around shared meals and outdoor activities. The locals engage in walking, dancing, and farming, fostering not only physical health but also emotional well-being. This social aspect reinforces the idea that physical activity is most beneficial when it is a communal experience, enhancing motivation and creating bonds that nurture mental health. These cultures remind us that integrating movement into our social lives can significantly elevate our overall quality of life.

The Maasai people of East Africa exemplify a culture where physical activity is not just a way to stay fit but also a vital component of their identity. Their traditional practices, including herding cattle and performing intricate dances, demand a high level of physical fitness and endurance. This active lifestyle is deeply embedded in their customs and rituals, showcasing how physical prowess is celebrated and respected. The Maasai demonstrate that physical activity can serve as a powerful expression of cultural heritage, infusing daily life with purpose and pride. By recognizing the role of cultural identity in physical activity, we can inspire ourselves to seek out and celebrate our own active traditions.

Furthermore, the concept of sustainable living is intricately linked to physical activity in many of the world's healthiest cultures. In Bhutan, where Gross National Happiness is prioritized over economic growth, the population engages in walking and hiking as primary modes of transportation. The breathtaking landscapes encourage outdoor activities that not only promote physical health but also cultivate a profound connection to nature. Such practices foster a sustainable lifestyle, where the health of the individual is aligned with the health of the environment. By embracing physical activity as part of a sustainable lifestyle, we can enhance our well-being while nurturing the planet.

Ultimately, the lessons from these active cultures reveal that physical activity is more than just exercise; it is a holistic approach to wellness that encompasses community, identity, and sustainability. By drawing inspiration from the practices of the healthiest populations, we can transform our own lifestyles. Incorporating movement into our daily routines, celebrating active traditions, and fostering connections through shared activities can lead to a healthier, more fulfilling life. As we embrace these lessons, we discover that wellness is not a destination but a journey enriched by the vibrant tapestry of cultures that surround us.

Nutrition: Eating Like the Healthiest People

Nutrition plays a crucial role in the lives of the healthiest people around the globe, transcending borders and cultural practices. These individuals often share a profound connection to their food, viewing it not merely as sustenance but as a vital component of their overall well-being. By exploring the culinary traditions of various cultures renowned for their healthful practices, we can uncover valuable lessons on how to nourish our bodies and minds. Embracing the principles of whole, unprocessed foods, seasonal eating, and local sourcing can significantly transform our relationship with food, leading to enhanced vitality and longevity.

In many cultures, traditional fermented foods take center stage as staples of their diets. From the tangy kimchi of Korea to the creamy kefir enjoyed in Eastern Europe, these probiotic-rich foods are celebrated for their ability to support gut health and boost immunity. The fermentation process not only preserves food but also enhances its nutritional profile, making it easier for our bodies to absorb essential nutrients. By integrating these ancient practices into our modern diets, we can cultivate a thriving gut microbiome that fosters overall health, showcasing the remarkable synergy between tradition and well-being.

Moreover, the practice of eating mindfully is prevalent among the healthiest populations. Instead of rushing through meals, they savor every bite, appreciating the flavors, textures, and aromas of their food. This approach fosters a deeper connection to what they consume, promoting better digestion and preventing overeating. Mindful eating encourages us to listen to our bodies and recognize hunger cues, allowing us to make more intentional choices that align with our health goals. By adopting this practice, we can cultivate a more harmonious relationship with food, transforming each meal into a nourishing ritual.

Sustainable living is another key aspect of the nutrition practices observed in the healthiest cultures. These communities prioritize local, seasonal ingredients that not only support their health but also benefit the environment. By choosing to eat foods that are grown and harvested within their ecosystems, they reduce their carbon footprint and promote biodiversity. This holistic approach to nutrition emphasizes the interconnectedness of personal well-being and the health of the planet. As we embrace sustainability in our diets, we can contribute to a healthier world while nourishing ourselves in the process.

Ultimately, the journey to eating like the healthiest people on earth involves a commitment to embracing diverse culinary traditions, prioritizing gut health through fermented foods, practicing mindful eating, and fostering sustainable habits. By drawing inspiration from cultures that have thrived for generations, we can create a rich tapestry of nutrition that not only enhances our physical health but also nurtures our mental and emotional well-being. The path to wellness is illuminated by the wisdom of those who came before us, inviting us to explore, experiment, and ultimately transform our lives through the power of food.

Community and Connection: The Power of Relationships

In the tapestry of human existence, the threads of community and connection stand out as some of the most vibrant and essential. Across the globe, cultures deeply rooted in relationships have demonstrated that the health of individuals often mirrors the health of their communities. From the bustling markets of Morocco to the serene villages of Okinawa, people thrive not just through individual pursuits but through the bonds they share with one another. These connections foster a sense of belonging and purpose, creating a fertile ground for emotional and physical well-being. When we prioritize relationships, we unlock a powerful source of resilience that can help us navigate life's challenges.

Traditional fermented foods, celebrated for their health benefits, also play a crucial role in fostering community connections. In many cultures, the preparation and sharing of these foods are communal activities that bring people together. Whether it's the vibrant kimchi of Korea or the tangy kefir from Eastern Europe, these foods are often made using time-honored recipes passed down through generations. The act of fermentation itself embodies the essence of collaboration, as beneficial bacteria thrive in environments where diverse elements come together. In this way, the act of creating and consuming fermented foods becomes a communal ritual that nurtures both gut health and social ties, reinforcing the idea that our well-being is intertwined with those around us.

Sustainable living practices, too, emphasize the importance of community and connection. Cultures that prioritize sustainable methods often do so through collective efforts, whether it's community gardens in urban areas or cooperative farming in rural settings. These practices not only reduce environmental footprints but also cultivate relationships among individuals sharing a common goal. The sense of unity that emerges fosters trust and cooperation, which are essential for both ecological and personal health. As communities engage in sustainable practices, they create a supportive network that empowers individuals to live healthier lives, enhancing both physical health and collective well-being.

The psychological benefits of strong relationships cannot be overstated. Research consistently shows that people with robust social connections experience lower levels of stress, anxiety, and depression. In cultures where collective gatherings, rituals, and celebrations are the norm, individuals find solace and strength in knowing they are not alone. The support networks formed through these connections offer not only emotional comfort but also practical assistance, reinforcing the idea that we are stronger together. As we explore the healthiest cultures globally, it becomes evident that their commitment to nurturing relationships is a cornerstone of their overall health and longevity.

Ultimately, the journey toward wellness is not just an individual endeavor but a communal one. By recognizing the profound impact that relationships have on our health, we can begin to cultivate a lifestyle that prioritizes connection. Whether through the shared enjoyment of traditional foods, the collective pursuit of sustainability, or simply the act of coming together, we can harness the power of community to enhance our well-being. In a world where isolation can often feel overwhelming, it is essential to remember that the bonds we forge with others are among the most powerful tools we have in our quest for a healthier, more fulfilling life.

Chapter 6: The Future of Global Wellness

Innovations in Health and Wellness

Innovations in health and wellness are reshaping our understanding of what it means to live a healthy life. Across the globe, cultures are merging traditional practices with modern science to create holistic approaches to wellness. This fusion is not only enhancing physical health but also nurturing mental and emotional well-being. As we explore the healthiest communities, we uncover a treasure trove of innovative practices that inspire us to rethink our lifestyles and embrace a more balanced way of living.

Traditional fermented foods have long been celebrated for their profound impact on gut health, an area that has recently gained immense attention in the wellness community. Cultures such as those in South Korea with their kimchi, or in Japan with miso and natto, have understood the importance of these foods for centuries. The fermentation process not only preserves nutrients but also introduces beneficial probiotics that support digestive health. As research continues to unveil the intricate relationship between gut health and overall wellness, these time-honored practices are experiencing a renaissance, inspiring individuals worldwide to incorporate these nutrient-dense foods into their diets.

Sustainable living stands at the forefront of innovations in health and wellness, emphasizing the interconnectedness of our environment and personal well-being. Communities that prioritize sustainable practices—such as organic farming, local sourcing, and minimal waste—are not only protecting the planet but also enhancing their residents' health. This approach fosters a sense of community and belonging, empowering individuals to take control of their health through conscious choices. By promoting a lifestyle that respects the earth, these cultures demonstrate how our choices can lead to a more vibrant, healthier life for both ourselves and future generations.

Incorporating innovative health technologies further enriches the wellness landscape. Wearable devices and health apps are revolutionizing how we track our health metrics, encouraging proactive health management. From monitoring physical activity to meditation practices, these tools empower individuals to take charge of their well-being. Combined with traditional wellness practices, such as mindfulness and yoga, technology becomes a valuable ally in our journey toward holistic health. This integration of old and new fosters a culture of continuous learning and adaptation, inspiring people to seek out what truly resonates with their personal wellness journey.

As we delve deeper into the innovations in health and wellness, we are reminded of the rich tapestry of traditions that span the globe. Each culture brings unique insights that can enhance our understanding of health, urging us to embrace diversity in our wellness practices. By learning from the healthiest communities, we not only enrich our own lives but also cultivate a global perspective on well-being. In this interconnected world, the innovations in health and wellness pave the way for a brighter, healthier future for all.

Bridging Traditional Knowledge and Modern Science

In an age where modern science dominates the conversation around health and wellness, the wisdom of traditional knowledge offers a profound counterbalance. Across the globe, indigenous cultures have cultivated a deep understanding of their environments, often relying on centuries-old practices that promote holistic well-being. This synergy between traditional knowledge and contemporary scientific research can illuminate pathways to healthier lifestyles, emphasizing the importance of sustainability and community-driven practices that nurture both the body and the planet.

Consider the vibrant world of traditional fermented foods, which has long been celebrated for its health benefits. Cultures from Asia to Africa have mastered the art of fermentation, turning simple ingredients into nutritional powerhouses. Kimchi, sauerkraut, and kefir are not merely culinary delights; they are living examples of how local traditions harness natural processes to enhance gut health. Modern science now validates these practices, revealing how probiotics in fermented foods support a balanced microbiome, boosting immunity and digestion. By bridging these two realms, we find a richer understanding of health that honors both time-tested wisdom and cutting-edge research.

Sustainable living is another crucial area where traditional practices and modern science intersect. Indigenous communities often thrive on principles of conservation and respect for nature, fostering relationships with their environment that prioritize long-term health over short-term gains. This holistic view is increasingly relevant in today's world, where climate change and environmental degradation pose significant threats to global health. By integrating sustainable practices—such as permaculture, natural medicine, and community gardens—into modern lifestyles, we can enhance our well-being while also protecting the ecosystems that support us.

The journey toward wellness is not just individual; it is inherently collective. Traditional cultures often emphasize community and shared responsibility, nurturing social bonds that contribute to mental and emotional health. In contrast, modern society has seen a rise in isolation and disconnection, which can hinder our overall well-being. By drawing inspiration from traditional social structures, we can foster connections that promote resilience, empathy, and support, ultimately leading to healthier communities. This communal approach to wellness is vital, as it recognizes that our health is intertwined with the health of those around us.

As we explore the healthiest cultures around the globe, it becomes clear that the fusion of traditional knowledge and modern science holds immense potential for transformation. This dynamic interplay encourages us to rethink our health paradigms, inviting innovative solutions that are both effective and sustainable. Embracing this holistic perspective not only honors the wisdom of our ancestors but also equips us to tackle contemporary health challenges with creativity and compassion. In this endeavor, we can cultivate a world where wellness is accessible, inclusive, and deeply rooted in the rich tapestry of human experience.

The Role of Technology in Promoting Wellness

In today's rapidly evolving world, technology plays a pivotal role in promoting wellness across diverse cultures. From wearable health monitors to telemedicine, the integration of technology into daily life has transformed how individuals approach their health and well-being. This shift is particularly evident in cultures renowned for their health practices, where technology complements traditional wisdom, creating a holistic approach to wellness. By harnessing the power of innovation, individuals can enhance their understanding of personal health, leading to more informed decisions that support longevity and vitality.

One of the most significant advancements in health technology is the rise of wearable devices, which empower users to track their physical activity, sleep patterns, and even dietary habits. In cultures where wellness is a communal value, these devices not only promote individual accountability but also foster a sense of community. For instance, in regions known for their active lifestyles, such as the Mediterranean, families and friends often share their fitness goals and achievements through apps, creating an encouraging environment that motivates everyone to stay active and healthy. This collective engagement underscores the importance of social support in maintaining wellness.

Moreover, the resurgence of interest in traditional fermented foods has been greatly aided by technology. With the advent of online platforms and social media, knowledge about the benefits of gut health and fermentation techniques has spread rapidly. Cultures that have long embraced these practices, such as those in East Asia and

Eastern Europe, are now sharing their time-honored recipes and methods with a global audience. This exchange not only revitalizes traditional diets but also promotes a deeper understanding of the microbiome's role in overall health. As more individuals explore the gut-brain connection, they are inspired to incorporate these nutrient-rich foods into their daily routines, enhancing their well-being.

Sustainable living is another area where technology fosters wellness by promoting eco-friendly practices and reducing environmental stressors. Smart homes equipped with energy-efficient appliances and water-saving technologies contribute to a healthier living environment. In cultures that prioritize sustainability, such as those in Scandinavian countries, technology is seamlessly integrated into everyday life, making it easier for individuals to adopt practices that support both their health and the planet. This dual focus on personal and environmental well-being creates a holistic approach to health that resonates with the growing global movement toward sustainability.

Finally, telemedicine has revolutionized access to healthcare, particularly in remote and underserved areas. This technology bridges the gap between patients and healthcare providers, ensuring that individuals can receive timely advice and treatment regardless of their location. In countries with vast geographic challenges, such as those in the Pacific Islands, telemedicine has become a lifeline for many, promoting preventative care and reducing the burden of chronic diseases. By making healthcare more accessible, technology empowers individuals to take charge of their health, reinforcing the idea that wellness is not only a personal journey but also a collective responsibility. As we embrace these technological advancements, we move closer to realizing a world where wellness is within everyone's reach.

Creating a Global Wellness Movement

Creating a global wellness movement requires a collective commitment to nurturing health in ways that transcend geographical boundaries. As we embark on this journey, it is vital to recognize that wellness is not a one-size-fits-all concept. Instead, it is a rich tapestry woven from the diverse practices, traditions, and beliefs of cultures around the world. By embracing these differences, we can cultivate a global community where wellness flourishes, drawing inspiration from the healthiest people across the globe and their unique approaches to living well.

One of the cornerstones of a global wellness movement lies in the appreciation of traditional fermented foods and their profound impact on gut health. Cultures such as those in Japan, Korea, and Eastern Europe have long understood the importance of these foods, which not only enhance flavor but also promote digestive health and overall vitality. By sharing knowledge about these practices and encouraging their incorporation into everyday diets, we can empower individuals to reconnect with their food sources and embrace the transformative benefits of fermentation. This revival of ancient wisdom serves not only to nourish bodies but also to strengthen communities through shared culinary experiences.

Sustainable living is another vital aspect of this movement, as it emphasizes the interconnectedness of our health and the health of our planet. Embracing sustainable practices fosters a sense of responsibility toward the environment, ensuring that future generations can enjoy the same resources we have today. By highlighting cultures that exemplify sustainable living—such as the indigenous practices of various communities or the permaculture methods employed in many parts of the world—we can inspire individuals to adopt eco-friendly habits. This commitment to sustainability not only enhances personal well-being but also contributes to the collective health of our global community.

As we create a global wellness movement, it is essential to foster a sense of inclusivity and accessibility. By sharing stories of resilience and wellness from around the world, we can inspire individuals from all walks of life to engage in their health journeys. Workshops, online platforms, and community gatherings can serve as powerful tools for education and connection, allowing people to learn from one another and embrace diverse wellness practices. By emphasizing the importance of community support, we can create a nurturing environment where everyone feels empowered to pursue their wellness goals.

Ultimately, the creation of a global wellness movement is about more than just individual health; it is about cultivating a sense of belonging and shared purpose. By coming together to celebrate the richness of our cultural heritages, we can foster a world where well-being is prioritized and valued. This collective effort will not only enhance our physical health but also enrich our emotional and spiritual lives, creating a brighter, healthier future for all. Through collaboration, education, and a commitment to sustainable practices, we can ignite a movement that transcends borders and inspires generations to come.

Chapter 7: Personal Journeys to Wellness

Testimonials from Around the World

In our journey through the tapestry of global cultures, the voices of individuals from diverse backgrounds resonate with shared wisdom about wellness. Testimonials from around the world reveal how local traditions, practices, and philosophies contribute to the health and vitality of communities. From the vibrant streets of Tokyo to the serene landscapes of the Peruvian Andes, people are embracing lifestyles that honor their heritage while promoting holistic well-being. These stories inspire us to reflect on our own habits and consider how we can incorporate elements of these thriving cultures into our lives.

In Japan, the concept of "Ikigai" embodies the intersection of passion, mission, vocation, and profession. This philosophy encourages individuals to find purpose in their daily activities, fostering a deep sense of fulfillment. Yuki, a 75-year-old woman from Kyoto, shares her journey of maintaining balance through practices like meditation, seasonal eating, and community engagement. Her testimony emphasizes that wellness transcends mere physical health; it is a harmonious blend of emotional and spiritual well-being. Yuki's story serves as a reminder that nurturing our sense of purpose can lead to a longer, more fulfilling life.

Moving across the globe to the Mediterranean region, we encounter the wisdom of traditional diets that have stood the test of time. Maria, a grandmother from a small village in Italy, recounts the importance of family meals centered around locally sourced, seasonal ingredients. Her enthusiasm for preparing dishes rich in vegetables, whole grains, and healthy fats reflects a deep-seated belief in the power of food to heal and connect. Maria's experiences underscore the significance of communal dining, not only for physical nourishment but also for cultivating relationships that enhance our emotional and psychological health.

In the heart of Africa, the embrace of traditional fermented foods presents another facet of wellness. Kwame, a health advocate from Ghana, passionately shares his journey of rediscovering the benefits of fermented staples like gari and kenkey. He highlights how these foods, rich in probiotics, support gut health and overall immunity. Kwame's testimony reveals a growing movement among young people in his community to return to ancestral practices that honor their roots while promoting modern health benefits. His words inspire us to explore the riches of fermented foods, recognizing their potential to enhance our gut health and resilience.

Finally, we turn to the wisdom of indigenous communities in South America, where sustainable living and deep respect for nature form the foundation of well-being. Ana, an elder from a Quechua community in the Andes, speaks passionately about the interconnectedness of all living things. Her commitment to sustainable farming practices and preserving biodiversity not only sustains her community but also fosters a profound sense of peace and belonging. Ana's insights remind us that our health is intricately linked to the health of our planet, encouraging us to adopt sustainable practices that honor both our bodies and the earth. These global testimonials, woven together, illustrate a rich mosaic of wellness that transcends borders and speaks to the universal human desire for health, connection, and purpose.

Learning from Cultural Differences

In our quest for wellness, one of the most profound lessons we can learn comes from immersing ourselves in the rich tapestry of diverse cultures around the globe. Each culture offers unique insights and practices that have been honed over centuries, revealing the intricate relationship between lifestyle, health, and happiness. By embracing cultural differences, we open ourselves to new ways of thinking about wellness, encouraging a holistic approach that harmonizes body, mind, and spirit. This journey of exploration not only enhances our understanding of health but also inspires us to integrate these diverse practices into our own lives.

Among the most fascinating aspects of cultural differences is the role traditional fermented foods play in promoting gut health. Cultures such as those in Japan, Korea, and the Mediterranean have long embraced fermented foods as staples of their diets. These foods are not merely culinary delights; they are vital for nurturing the microbiome, which is increasingly recognized as a cornerstone of overall health. By learning from these cultures, we can appreciate the importance of incorporating fermented foods like kimchi, miso, and yogurt into our diets, fostering a thriving gut flora that can lead to improved digestion, enhanced immunity, and greater emotional well-being.

Sustainable living practices also shed light on the interconnectedness of health and the environment. Cultures that prioritize sustainable practices often experience lower stress levels and a stronger sense of community. For example, the indigenous peoples of various regions employ methods of agriculture that respect the land and its resources, promoting not just their health but that of future generations. By observing and adopting these sustainable practices, we can cultivate a lifestyle that not only benefits our personal well-being but also contributes to the health of our planet. This symbiotic relationship between nature and our well-being serves as a powerful reminder that taking care of the earth is integral to taking care of ourselves.

Furthermore, learning from cultural differences encourages us to challenge our assumptions about health and wellness. In many cultures, the concept of wellness extends beyond the physical to encompass emotional and spiritual dimensions. For instance, practices like mindfulness in Buddhist cultures or the emphasis on family and community in many African societies highlight the importance of mental and emotional health. By embracing these broader definitions, we can create a more inclusive understanding of wellness, one that recognizes the importance of emotional resilience, social connections, and spiritual fulfillment in our overall health.

Ultimately, the wisdom derived from cultural differences offers us a rich reservoir of knowledge to draw upon as we navigate our personal wellness journeys. By actively seeking to understand and incorporate the best practices from around the world, we empower ourselves to create a lifestyle that embraces diversity and promotes holistic health. This journey is not just about individual well-being; it is about fostering a global community rooted in respect, understanding, and a shared commitment to wellness. As we learn from one another, we become not only healthier individuals but also more compassionate global citizens.

Transforming Challenges into Opportunities

In the journey toward wellness, challenges often emerge as defining moments that shape our paths. Across cultures, those who have faced adversity have frequently transformed their struggles into opportunities for growth and betterment. This alchemy of turning hardships into stepping stones is evident in the daily lives of the healthiest communities around the globe. By embracing challenges as catalysts for change, individuals and societies can cultivate resilience, foster innovation, and ultimately achieve a deeper sense of well-being.

Take the example of traditional fermented foods, a cornerstone of gut health in many cultures. In regions where food scarcity or poor nutritional options prevail, communities have turned to fermentation as a means of preservation and enhancement of food quality. This practice not only ensures the longevity of food supplies but also enriches diets with probiotics and essential nutrients. By transforming the challenge of limited resources into a solution that promotes health, these cultures exemplify how adversity can lead to the discovery of beneficial practices that endure through generations.

Sustainable living also highlights the transformative power of challenges. In areas grappling with environmental degradation, communities have recognized the urgent need to innovate and adapt. By embracing sustainable practices, such as permaculture and organic farming, they have not only addressed ecological concerns but also enhanced their overall well-being. This shift towards sustainability is not merely a response to a crisis; it is an opportunity to create healthier environments, both physically and mentally. The result is a profound connection to nature and a renewed appreciation for the resources that sustain life.

Moreover, the journey of wellness is often marked by individual stories of triumph over personal challenges. From overcoming health issues to breaking free from societal constraints, individuals who embrace their struggles can inspire others to do the same. These narratives serve as powerful reminders that wellness is not just a destination but a continuous journey shaped by our ability to navigate life's hurdles. The stories of those who have transformed their challenges into opportunities illuminate pathways for others, encouraging a collective movement toward a healthier world.

Ultimately, the art of transforming challenges into opportunities is a universal theme that resonates across cultures. It is a testament to the human spirit's capacity for resilience and innovation. By learning from the practices and philosophies of the healthiest people around the globe, we can all cultivate a mindset that views challenges as gateways to growth. Embracing this perspective not only enhances our individual well-being but also fosters a global community that thrives on shared knowledge and mutual support, leading to a healthier, more sustainable future for all.

Inspiring Change in Your Own Life

Inspiring change in your own life begins with the recognition that transformation is possible and within your grasp. Embracing a mindset open to new possibilities can set the stage for profound shifts. All around the world, cultures have thrived by adopting practices that promote wellness, whether through traditional diets, community engagement, or sustainable living. By observing and integrating these elements into your daily routine, you can cultivate a life that aligns with your health goals, fostering both personal growth and a deeper connection to the planet.

One of the most powerful ways to inspire change is by exploring traditional fermented foods, which have long been the cornerstone of many healthy cultures. From miso in Japan to kimchi in Korea, these foods not only nourish the body but also support gut health, which is increasingly recognized as fundamental to overall well-being. By incorporating these nutrient-dense foods into your diet, you can enhance your digestive health, boost your immune system, and even improve your mental clarity. Start small by adding a serving of fermented vegetables or a probiotic-rich drink to your meals. This simple act can lead to a cascade of positive changes in how you feel physically and mentally.

Sustainable living is another transformative avenue that can inspire change in your life. The practices of cultures that prioritize sustainability—like the Mediterranean diet, which emphasizes plant-based foods and local sourcing—encourage a harmonious relationship with the environment. By adopting similar habits, such as shopping at local farmers' markets or growing your own herbs and vegetables, you not only improve your diet but also contribute positively to the planet. This commitment to sustainability fosters a sense of purpose and connection, enriching your life as you become more mindful of the impact your choices have on the world around you.

Engaging with your community can also serve as a catalyst for personal transformation. Many of the world's healthiest cultures emphasize the importance of social connections, which are vital for emotional health and resilience. By participating in community events, volunteering, or simply spending time with loved ones, you create a network of support that can help you navigate life's challenges. This social engagement not only enhances your happiness but also encourages accountability in your wellness journey, motivating you to stick to the positive changes you wish to see in your life.

Ultimately, inspiring change in your own life is about taking actionable steps towards a healthier, more fulfilling existence. By integrating traditional fermented foods, adopting sustainable practices, and fostering meaningful connections, you create a life that reflects your values and aspirations. Remember, every small change contributes to a greater impact, and as you embark on this journey, you not only transform your own life but also inspire those around you to embrace wellness in their own unique ways. Embrace the journey with enthusiasm and an open heart, knowing that the path to wellness is one filled with endless possibilities.

Chapter 8: Conclusion: A Global Perspective on Health

Embracing Diversity in Wellness Practices

Embracing diversity in wellness practices is essential as we navigate a world rich in traditions, cultures, and health philosophies. Each culture offers unique insights into maintaining well-being, revealing that there is no singular path to health. By exploring various wellness practices from around the globe, we can appreciate the myriad ways people nurture their bodies, minds, and spirits. This exploration encourages us to celebrate differences and uncover holistic approaches that resonate with our individual needs.

Traditional fermented foods serve as a powerful testament to the integration of cultural heritage and health. From the tangy taste of kimchi in Korea to the probiotic-rich sauerkraut in Germany, these foods exemplify how communities have long understood the importance of gut health. Fermentation is not merely a method of preservation; it is a ritual that connects people to their land and history. By incorporating these time-honored practices into our diets, we can enhance our gut microbiome, fostering immunity and overall wellness. This melding of tradition and nutrition invites us to experiment and embrace diverse flavors that nourish our bodies in profound ways.

Sustainable living emerges as another cornerstone of holistic wellness, deeply intertwined with the health of our planet and ourselves. Cultures that prioritize sustainability often exhibit remarkable well-being, showcasing the interconnectedness of environmental health and personal vitality. Indigenous practices around the world highlight the wisdom of living in harmony with nature. From permaculture in Australia to the communal farming methods in Africa, these approaches teach us that our health is inextricably linked to the health of our ecosystems. By adopting sustainable practices in our own lives, we not only support the planet but also cultivate a sense of purpose and belonging.

The embrace of diverse wellness practices also encourages a broader understanding of mental and emotional health. Cultures utilize various forms of mindfulness, meditation, and community engagement to foster resilience and emotional balance. For instance, the practice of yoga, originating from ancient India, offers not only physical benefits but also profound mental clarity and emotional healing. Similarly, communal gatherings and storytelling traditions found in many cultures highlight the importance of connection and shared experiences in promoting mental well-being. By incorporating these diverse practices into our daily lives, we can support our mental health and create a more compassionate world.

Ultimately, embracing diversity in wellness practices enriches our understanding of health and well-being. It inspires us to step outside our comfort zones, exploring the wisdom of other cultures while integrating their teachings into our unique journeys. By celebrating these differences, we not only enhance our personal wellness but also contribute to a global tapestry of health that honors the varied experiences of humanity. As we embark on this journey, let us remain open to the lessons that diverse practices offer, recognizing that in our collective quest for wellness, we are stronger together.

The Path Forward: Collective Responsibility

In an interconnected world where our actions ripple across borders, the concept of collective responsibility emerges as a guiding principle for wellness. The health of individuals is inextricably linked to the health of communities and ecosystems. As we strive to uncover the healthiest cultures around the globe, we must recognize that the path forward requires us to embrace this interconnectedness, cultivating a sense of shared responsibility for our collective well-being. This journey is not only about personal health choices but also about fostering environments where sustainable practices flourish and where traditional wisdom is honored and integrated into modern lifestyles.

Traditional fermented foods, celebrated for their profound impact on gut health, are a testament to the wisdom of our ancestors. These age-old practices reflect a deep understanding of the symbiotic relationship between humans and nature. As we witness a resurgence of interest in these foods, we are reminded that the knowledge of preparing and consuming them belongs to communities that have thrived for generations. By supporting local artisans and farmers who prioritize traditional methods, we not only enhance our own health but also empower entire communities. This collective effort to preserve and promote healthy cultural practices fosters a vibrant tapestry of wellness that transcends individual gain.

Sustainable living emerges as another critical facet of our shared responsibility. The choices we make regarding food, energy, and waste not only affect our personal health but also have far-reaching implications for the planet. By adopting practices that prioritize sustainability, we can contribute to healthier ecosystems that, in turn, nurture our well-being. Simple actions, such as supporting local agriculture or reducing plastic consumption, can lead to significant positive changes. When we come together as a global community, advocating for sustainable practices, we pave the way for future generations to inherit a healthier world, rich in resources and biodiversity.

Moreover, community engagement plays a pivotal role in fostering a wellness culture. By creating spaces where individuals can share knowledge, experiences, and resources, we nurture a sense of belonging that is essential for mental and emotional well-being. Collective events, whether they are workshops on traditional cooking methods or community gardens, serve as platforms for connection and collaboration. These gatherings not only celebrate diverse cultures but also emphasize the importance of working together toward common goals. When we invest in our communities, we strengthen the fabric of society, allowing wellness to flourish in a supportive environment.

As we embark on this journey towards collective responsibility, let us be inspired by the healthiest cultures around the world. Their commitment to wellness, sustainability, and community underscores the profound impact of interconnected actions. By embracing our role as stewards of both our health and our planet, we can create a future where wellness is not a solitary pursuit but a shared endeavor. Together, we can cultivate a world that honors tradition, promotes sustainable practices, and fosters a collective sense of responsibility—ensuring that the path forward is not just about individual health, but about the thriving of all.

Your Role in the Global Wellness Community

Your participation in the global wellness community is not just a personal journey; it is a transformative experience that resonates far beyond individual borders. As you explore the healthiest cultures around the world, you become part of a larger narrative that emphasizes the interconnectedness of health, environment, and tradition. By understanding and embracing diverse approaches to wellness, you cultivate a mindset that appreciates the richness of different lifestyles and practices. This journey allows you to not only enhance your own well-being but also contribute to a collective movement that values health on a global scale.

Engaging with traditional fermented foods is an excellent way to deepen your connection to the global wellness community. These foods, cherished across various cultures, hold the key to gut health, which is increasingly recognized as vital to overall well-being. By incorporating fermented foods into your diet, you honor ancient practices while supporting your body's microbiome. This simple act of eating becomes a bridge between you and cultures that have thrived on these nutritious staples for generations. Sharing recipes, stories, and experiences with others fosters a sense of unity and encourages knowledge exchange, reinforcing the idea that health is a communal endeavor.

Sustainable living plays a pivotal role in enhancing both personal and communal wellness. By adopting eco-friendly practices, you contribute to a healthier planet, which in turn supports healthier communities. Understanding how local ecosystems impact health and well-being empowers you to make choices that benefit not just yourself, but also the environment and future generations. Whether it's reducing waste, supporting local agriculture, or participating in community gardens, every action you take reverberates throughout the global wellness network. Your commitment to sustainability demonstrates a profound respect for the interdependence of all living beings, fostering a culture of care and responsibility.

As you navigate your role within this community, consider how sharing your journey can inspire others. Your experiences, whether in discovering the benefits of traditional wellness practices or advocating for sustainable living, can spark conversations that lead to greater awareness and action. Social media platforms, local gatherings, and wellness workshops are powerful avenues for storytelling. By sharing the knowledge you've gained, you not only amplify your voice but also encourage a ripple effect of positive change. Every story has the potential to ignite curiosity and motivate others to embark on their own wellness journeys, creating a vibrant tapestry of shared experiences.

Ultimately, your role in the global wellness community is a testament to the power of collective action. By embracing diverse traditions, advocating for sustainable practices, and sharing your experiences, you contribute to a movement that champions health and well-being for all. The journey is not solely about individual improvement; it is about weaving together the threads of cultures, practices, and beliefs to create a healthier world. Together, we can cultivate a global culture of wellness that celebrates the richness of human experience and the beauty of our shared commitment to a healthier future.